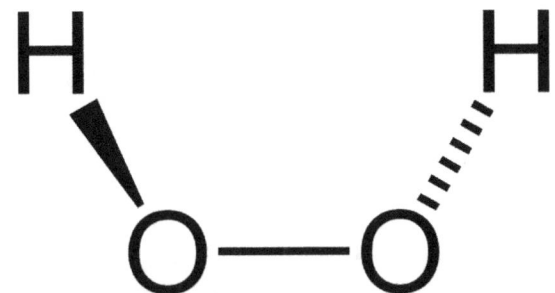

Hydrogen Peroxide:

Discover The Amazing Health Benefits And Many Uses Of This Natural Compound

By Julie Kingston

Disclaimer and Terms of Use:

Effort has been made to ensure that the information in this book is accurate and complete, however, the author and the publisher do not warrant the accuracy of the information, text and graphics contained within the book due to the rapidly changing nature of science, research, known and unknown facts and internet. The Author and the publisher do not hold any responsibility for errors, omissions or contrary interpretation of the subject matter herein. This book is presented solely for motivational and informational purposes only.

1. Table of Contents

2. What Hydrogen Peroxide Is

Hydrogen peroxide is a common household cleaning agent. It is basically a clear, heavy unstable compound with formidable oxidizing properties. Through oxidation, it is able to act on germs and deodorize the home. Hydrogen peroxide can be found in many forms but the best should be purchased from the pharmaceutical stores.

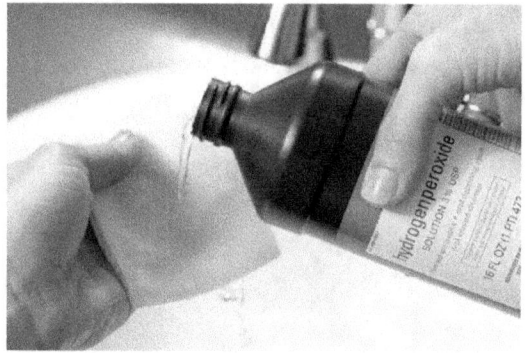

Hydrogen peroxide is the only germicide composed of water and oxygen, which makes it very safe for use around the home and the environment. It basically kills disease organisms by controlled burning, and is thus considered the world's safest sanitizer. Industrially, the compound is used in disinfection and bleaching thus underlining the unique features of the compound that make it the ideal cleaning agent.

Hydrogen peroxide has the formula H_2O_2 which is basically a water molecule with an additional atom of oxygen. Due to this extra oxygen atom, H_2O_2 is highly unstable and readily degenerates to water and oxygen or oxidizes anything in sight. The chemical's oxidizing properties make it an ideal disinfectant or cleaning agent because it practically burns out all bacteria in contact with it

Due to safety concerns though, hydrogen peroxide is shipped as an aqueous solution in water, mostly 35% by mass. Higher concentrations of the chemical have proved to be dangerous in the past. Actually, to correctly visualize how dangerous concentrated hydrogen peroxide can be, consider the fact that its used to propel rockets without the need of fuel. Just the steam and the thrust produced by the degenerating compound is enough.

One of the most attractive features of hydrogen peroxide as a cleaning agent is the fact that it is natural. H_2O_2 is formed naturally and can be found in the body especially in the respiratory tract and the blood. It is used by the body to fight bacterial infection and to kill off internal microbes.

Hydrogen peroxide is also occasionally produced naturally when the Ozone layer reacts with water vapor in the atmosphere in the presence of UV light. The result is always pure but very unstable quantities of a peroxide solution. This solution is very useful to mother earth because it serves as a natural cleanser of the atmosphere and the earth. From the sky downwards, if it falls on the ground it cleanses the fauna and flora. In the atmosphere, it may also react with harmful gases, to form less harmful substances. This goes to show just how much the wonder chemical fits into the earth's ecosystem.

The history of the compound dates back to 1818, when it was discovered by a French chemist. Hydrogen peroxide remains unstable and in case of heat, it is bound to explode in a thermal decomposition process.

Availability

As expected, hydrogen peroxide is available in aqueous solutions that are readily purchasable from multiple shops and outlets. You can either buy it from any chemist, pharmaceutical store or grocery stores. However, make sure that whatever you buy is standard food grade H_2O_2. Food grade here means that the chemical is fit for human consumption or ingestion. Note that any other variation of hydrogen peroxide is very harmful to your health. The reason is very simple. Due to the fact that hydrogen peroxide is highly unstable, manufacturers add stabilizers to it to prevent disintegration into water and oxygen.

Food grade hydrogen peroxide thus becomes tedious to handle and ship for manufacturers and is twice as expensive. However, though more expensive the cost will be very minimal compared to the common cleaning agents, disinfectants and oxidizing agents that can be used in place of hydrogen peroxide. At the end of the day, going for pure hydrogen peroxide will pay off. The pharmaceutical consumer grade is available in either 6% or 3% concentration by weight.

Traditional Uses of Hydrogen Peroxide

Industrially, hydrogen peroxide is used as bleach for paper in pulp industries. It is also used to make mild bleaches in the laundry industry at the same time. The chemical is also used in the purification of water from impurities during water treatment. In hospitals and biological research, hydrogen peroxide is used in medical disinfection. Chlorine based bleaches and disinfectant are cheaper but harmful to the environment and sometimes dangerous

Generally, dilute hydrogen peroxide is non-toxic to use at home and on the body. It is however important to note that the only grade that can be used at the home safely and naturally is the food grade hydrogen peroxide. You will find 35% as the highest concentration that can be sold to consumers and can be shipped. Note that hydrogen peroxide cannot be shipped by mail though. The variety you buy has to be approved by the U.S. food and drug administration department as well as the food and agriculture department.

3. Grades of Hydrogen Peroxide

Being a very sensitive reagent, the version of hydrogen peroxide you buy can be lethal or in effective, depending on your intended use. This brings in the question, is there any definite grading system for hydrogen peroxide. Well, grading H_2O_2 is a complex process since it can have various approaches. We are going to explore the two approaches of classifying the chemical or grading it so that you can be prepared for any jargon you encounter on your first purchase at the store. The first approach will involve the empirical logic behind technical names given to various brands and concentrations of hydrogen peroxide. The second way of classification will entail what you may actually find in the stores and what the various differences are.

i)   Ways of classifying hydrogen peroxide

As mentioned, this method will make you conversant with every approach chemists and biologists too have used to differentiate various grades of hydrogen peroxide. There are three major ways of classifying the chemical:

a) By percentage weight or volume

One of the most common descriptions you will encounter about hydrogen peroxide goes something like, "50% by weight, 35% by weight etc. What does this mean though? The simplest explanation is that the percentage given is the proportion of the hydrogen peroxide when weight is considered. The percentage would give you the amount of pure hydrogen peroxide you can find in each ration. For instance 500g of 50% H_2O_2 will contain exactly pure 250g H_2O_2 while the rest is distilled water. The water may also have small quantities of stabilizers and probably impurities meant to make the chemical have longer shelf life.

Proportionate volume descriptions are the same, as the weight and mass descriptions. The whole idea is that the given proportion is the actual amount of H_2O_2 you will expect to find in the mixtures. 35% H_2O_2 by volume contains only 350ml of pure H_2O_2 in every liter. Notice that volume will use liters as the bench mark while mass will use weight as the bench mark. The difference is always small though since the density of hydrogen peroxide is almost equal to that of water.

b) Commercial and food grade hydrogen peroxide

Due to the unstable nature of Hydrogen Peroxide, manufacturers prefer to introduce stabilizers to keep it stable, or non-volatile. Stabilizers are compounds that help keep the reactivity and decomposition down. This means that the hydrogen peroxide will only react in very compelling situations only. Compelling states would include exposure to ultraviolet light or the sun and heat. On normal circumstances, stabilized hydrogen peroxide will only decompose by 2% every year, which is commendable.

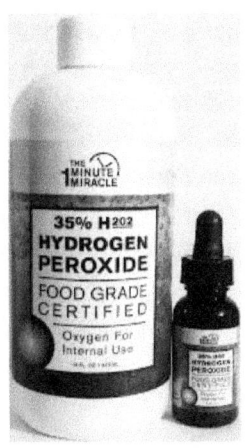

For commercially usable H_2O_2 this stabilization process is pretty much okay. It involves the addition of very dangerous chemicals that keep the chemical stable. This is in addition to bringing down the explosion risk during transit, as well as reducing the packaging hazards. This will naturally bring down the cost of the chemical to very low prices that are commercially viable. Commercial grade examples include HYPROX and OXTERIL.

Food grade hydrogen peroxide on the other hand, refers to the hydrogen peroxide with minimal quantities of stabilizers and sometimes none at all. It is very pure but also comes in very low concentrations often below 5% and a matching decomposition risk. This is mostly worth it if the hydrogen peroxide will end up in food. The stabilizers are dangerous chemicals known to cause diseases such as cancer and severe fluid disorders and thus any hydrogen peroxide that may be used at home should be strictly food grade, to avoid these. Apart from accidental direct ingestion, hydrogen peroxide stabilizers may also be taken in as residue after say cleaning a kitchen surface or cutting board, so keep off commercial hydrogen peroxide as much as possible.

c) By decomposition rate

Some manufacturers will care to classify their products in all possible ways, so it is likely that you will encounter a version of hydrogen peroxide classified by decomposition rate. This may be a little complicated for those with minimal chemistry knowledge, so I will put it in the simplest terms possible. Remember the only reason I am placing this here is because you will have to encounter the jargon at some point so it is good to know upfront to avoid confusion.

5% decomposition rate hydrogen peroxide means that only 5% of the original concentration will be lost when the solution is subjected to 96 degrees Celsius for 16 hours. The 16 hours at a particular temperature is a chemical standard for determining decomposition but you really don't have to remember that. Just keep the figure in mind, it is pretty consistent. A good example is a 5% rated sample of 50% hydrogen peroxide. This will result to 47.5% hydrogen peroxide after the exposure to the standard conditions. The simple idea in this third way of classifying is to know just how volatile a version of hydrogen peroxide is. Normally, the higher the decomposition rate, the better it is for home use, as this implies lower concentrations of stabilizers.

The second method of classifying is what you will most likely find at sale points. It is important to know the options you have so that you can buy the right grade, from the start.

ii)   Common grades found in grocery stores

This second classification is really not a way of classification, but a snapshot of the stuff you will find on the shelves of stores. Most manufacturers target the laymen when packaging and selling the chemical for retail. For this reason, the primary use of each bottle you encounter will most likely be printed on its sides. Below are some of the types you encounter.

a) 3.5% Pharmaceutical grade

If you go buying at a pharmaceutical store, chances are that this is the version you will encounter. A lot of people use it for first aid and doctors use it to sterilize medical paraphernalia. You can also find it in grocery stores at the first aid section. Make sure you read the package well. The 3.5% pharmaceutical grade can be used for bleaching hair, as well as disinfecting pools and baths. However, it is not recommended for internal uses, and much less not for home use. This make most likely has a great deal of stabilizers, which makes it unfit for use in the house. Some of the dangerous stabilizers found in pharmaceutical hydrogen peroxide include, acetanilide, Sodium Stanate, Phenol and Tetrasodium Phosphate. For this reason, use this for external procedures only or better still avoid it all together.

b) 6% beautician grade

For the grocery store or beauty shop buyer, this may be the version you encounter. The 6% beautician grade is a more highly concentrated version of the chemical. As expected it contains the dangerous stabilizers. This may be due to the fact that it is sold for use on hair alone as well as other beauty procedures. Do not use this for any other purpose. In a perfect setting, any discerning buyer would avoid it altogether.

c) 30% reagent grade

The reagent grade is slightly more concentrated. It can be found in grocery stores as well. Being the most common version around, you will find in virtually any academic institution, as well as office and school supplies. The reagent grade is used for various chemical reactions and lab experiments and demonstrations by students. Again, do not go for this one, it will be counterproductive. If you try to use it anywhere in your home, you may run into unprecedented trouble, dealing with stabilizers.

d) 30 to 32% Electronic grade

Another common place to find hydrogen peroxide is in electronics supply stores. Hydrogen peroxide is commonly used to clean electronic parts due to its unique set of qualities. You may use this to do electronics cleaning but the best version for multi-purpose hydrogen peroxide is actually the food grade. That means if you are not using the chemical on electronics, resist the temptation to buy this one too.

e) 35% food grade

Finally, there is the food grade hydrogen peroxide that comes at 35% concentration by weight. This is a version of hydrogen peroxide with minimal stabilizers. It is generally unstable and is packed in special containers that are able to stand the eventuality of a reaction. The food grade version is expensive; often more than twice the normal price but it is worth it if you plan to use it at home. The reason for its high price is apparent. Since there are no stabilizers, packaging, selling and distributing the product as it is always tedious and dangerous. For this reason, manufacturers have to cover up for the extra risk by charging a higher markup. The containers used to carry this one have to be strong and dark to mitigate any explosion risk.

The 35% food grade hydrogen peroxide may also be diluted by resale merchants, so look out for concentrations as low as 1% hydrogen peroxide. The important issue here is really not the concentration but the grade and the absence of impurities. This grade is used industrially to sanitize food packaging and food handling machinery. Food processors often spray it on the surface of food packaging to kill any microorganisms. For this reason, there has to be some regulation. The used food grade version has to be approved in the U.S. and must be certified by the United States department of Agriculture for use in preserving and sterilizing food.

Approval in this case will mean that the U. S. federal department has tested and certified that the hydrogen peroxide does not contain any harmful stabilizers as in the industrial standard. It also means each drum has been tested and approved to have the right concentration of the chemical as indicated in the packing. 35% hydrogen peroxide should for instance be pure 35% hydrogen peroxide without unnecessary dilution as some unscrupulous suppliers do.

Note that any other grade of hydrogen peroxide is very harmful when ingested and the only one fit for consumption is the "food grade". Remember there is no legal standard for "technical grade", and it could mean anything depending on the manufacturer. In this book, it is strongly recommended that you use food grade hydrogen peroxide for ALL the tricks that hydrogen peroxide can do for you in your home. There is really no need to try to better your life using a poisoned version of hydrogen peroxide, so be very careful at purchase, or abandon the home tips if you cannot locate food grade peroxide.

4. How to use Hydrogen Peroxide safely

With that solid introduction to the nature and blends of hydrogen peroxide, it is now appropriate to explore ways you can employ to ensure its safe to use around the home. Being an unstable liquid, there are numerous safety concerns in using hydrogen peroxide around the home and it is important to highlight some of them here to ensure you are safe at all times.

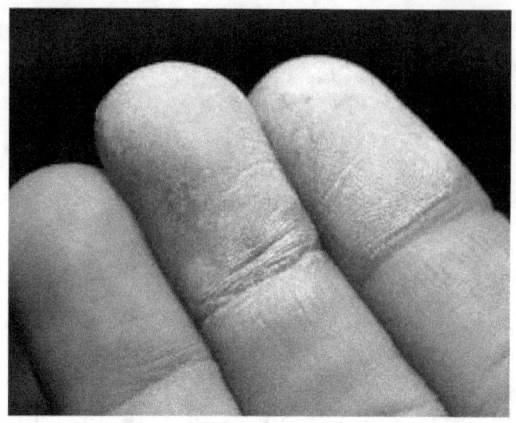

Below are some quick tips that will keep you safe with hydrogen peroxide in sight.

First, always dilute hydrogen peroxide for immediate consumption. One of the biggest mistakes that people commit is to dilute huge quantities of the chemical and store it. Remember you cannot store it as well as the original package. Diluting will generally introduce small impurities that will in effect weaken the chemical even before use. Remember it is also easier for your family to keep track of a small bottle of hydrogen peroxide than a huge bucket of diluted and unlabeled liquid.

Use distilled water in it if you have to dilute your hydrogen peroxide. If you cannot access distilled water or distill yourself, get battery water in the process. It will be as good as what you distill. Using tap water is a big no with hydrogen peroxide. Apart from the possibility of reacting with too many impurities, the hydrogen peroxide may oxidize chlorine and other ions in the water to form dangerous gas emissions.

When storing hydrogen peroxide for a long time or transporting it in hot weather, watch out for a bulge of storage containers. This may be a sign of too much decomposition and a possibility of explosion. Note that an increase in temperature of the solution would also mean that the chemical is undergoing rapid decomposition. Continuous bubbling indicates the container is unfit for keeping the hydrogen peroxide and it may be reacting with the chemical.

Beware of storing hydrogen peroxide in ordinary plastic containers, as it may rip them off. Remember that the plastic hydrogen peroxide is shipped in is special and may not be the one you find in your house. To be safe in the home, only use glass, stainless steel and pure aluminum to store your hydrogen peroxide. Pyrex glass is highly recommended. In case of high temperatures or bulging of your plastic storage container, change to a glass container or try to cool the container. Sustained high temperatures should immediately send alarm bells to dispose the hydrogen peroxide or dilute it further to manageable proportions.

Finally, as an important precaution, keep hydrogen peroxide out of the reach of kids. They may scar themselves in the process of playing around with the chemical. Kids tend to think anything that looks like water is edible, and you do not want that to happen to your kids. In case of accidental contact with skin, splash it with clean water to soothe the burn. You may store your hydrogen peroxide in a refrigerator but do not freeze it. With these straight forward guidelines, no ugly incidents will occur in your home when it comes to hydrogen peroxide.

How to dilute hydrogen peroxide safely

One of the biggest safety blunders hydrogen peroxide users do has everything to do with proper dilution. The wrong dilution ratio may mean a huge disservice to your skin or property. Note that hydrogen peroxide is a corrosive and hugely oxidizing agent that will readily consume anything in sight. This will be more so when in high concentrations. Below is a detailed guide on how to dilute hydrogen peroxide so that it can serve your safe usage intentions.

High concentrations of hydrogen peroxide can result in fire when in contact with some plastics and wood so you have to be careful when diluting. It is always prudent to add hydrogen peroxide into the water as opposed to the reverse. If you place pure hydrogen peroxide in a container that cannot handle its concentration, you may not love the result.

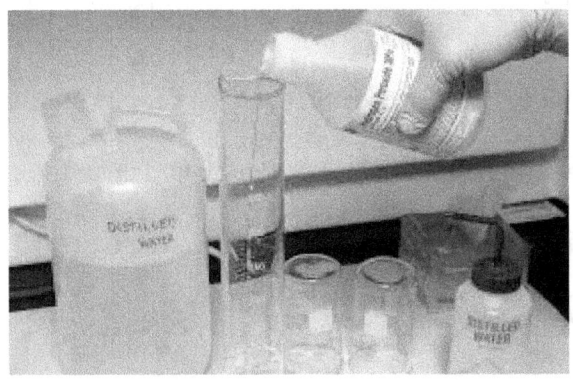

When using the compound, be sure to use it on an inconspicuous surface. Do not for instance test a wooden table from the top. Try cleaning the sides or a hidden area and monitor the reaction. If it cleans the hidden part without any incidence, you can then turn to the visible parts.

Make sure you dilute with distilled water only. Hydrogen peroxide reacts with anything impure in sight and it may not work well with tap or bottled water. Remember it will not only react, but it may result in some potentially dangerous salts such as sulfates and chlorates when mixed with tap water. Bottled water is also not suitable for diluting hydrogen peroxide. Stick to diluted water.

If you think your water is pure after all, (for whatever reason) it may be good to confirm with the TDS handy kit. The total dissolved solids device will give you a huge indication of the purity level of the water. The higher the TDS index, the less appropriate it is for use with hydrogen peroxide.

When diluting, always avoid skin contact or eye contact. Be sure to wear protective gloves and goggles before attempting to open the bottle. Always use a clean Pyrex glass to mix and measure out everything in the correct quantity.

Since most food grade hydrogen peroxide comes at 35% concentration, we will review the dilution dynamics using 35% concentration as a bench mark. Most of the hacks you do with hydrogen peroxide will require 3% concentration. When diluting it to 3% from 35%, measure it out with water in the ratio of 1:11. That is to mean 11 parts of distilled water should mix with 1 part of 35% hydrogen peroxide.

In case you want to bring up to 6% for beauty uses, you will need to double the ration of hydrogen peroxide. Mix 11 parts of distilled water with 2 parts of 35% hydrogen peroxide and you will have your 6% ration.

Finally remember to only mix what you will readily use as the more exposed the chemical is the more it will vaporize. Remember that hydrogen peroxide is highly sensitive to UV light and it may easily

decompose to water and Oxygen without introduction of any other

chemical, so keep it hidden. The remaining untouched hydrogen peroxide

should be kept in its original package. The packs again are specially

designed to withstand decomposition. Finally, though glass is safe to store

hydrogen peroxide in, it is brittle so it is recommended that you stick to

the plastic packaging due to a lower breaking risk.

5. Cleaning Uses Around The Home

Due to its strong oxidizing nature, hydrogen peroxide has many uses

around the home. Most of these uses involve cleaning and disinfecting

various parts of the home, from the bathroom to the kitchen. Remember

there is really nothing to fear if you are using food grade hydrogen

peroxide, so feel free to transform your home in the following ways.

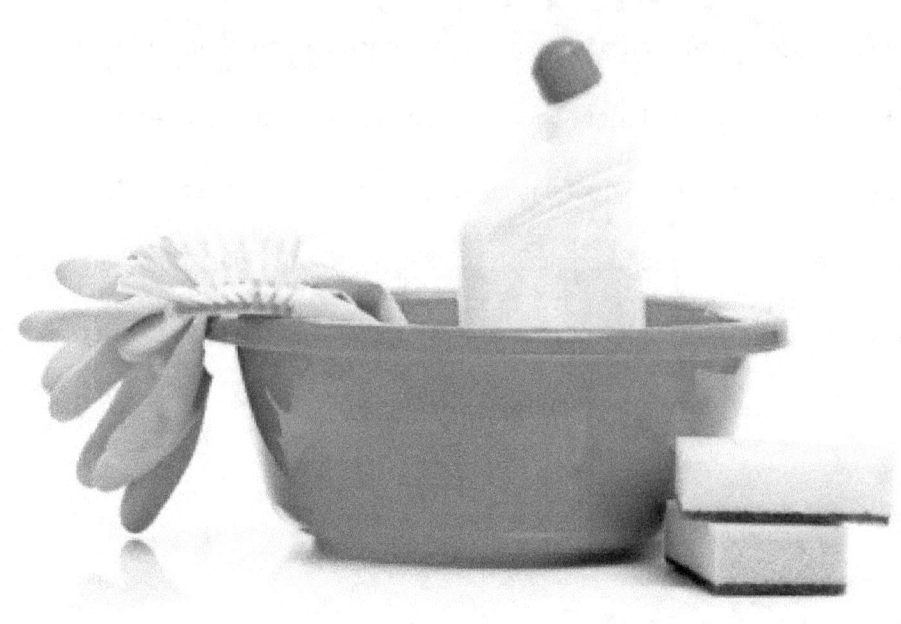

Whiten your clothes and remove stubborn stains with hydrogen peroxide

Hydrogen peroxide will readily bleach your whites to make them even whiter. Many types of bleach are based on hypochloric acid, which has a temporal effect. Well, hydrogen peroxide will do the job and leave the glow permanent. To do this, add a cup of hydrogen peroxide to your wash water to whiten your clothes. It is also a very great remedy for natural stains such as blood, sweat and wine on clothes and carpets, so feel free to use it even on stained non-whites. For blood stains, pour the liquid directly on the spot and let it sit for some seconds. Rub and rinse and iterate the process until the stain is completely gone.

Clean your surfaces with hydrogen peroxide

One wonderful feature of hydrogen peroxide is that it is antibacterial, antiviral as well as antifungal. With these amazing qualities in one substance, you can clean your kitchen counters and table tops with hydrogen peroxide, as well as every conceivable habitat for household microbes. The effect of hydrogen peroxide is that it will kill all the germs while leaving a fresh smell in the kitchen. All you need to do is to spray 3% hydrogen peroxide directly onto the affected areas and wipe off with a clean rag. Hydrogen peroxide will also readily loosen burn marks on your pans, so you can feel as creative as you want in the kitchen.

Sanitize your bedding

Bedding is hard to clean. Let's face it, even with a cleaning machine, there are stubborn stains that are found in sheets as well as blankets that rarely go away. Duvets and mattresses may exhibit a certain kind of pungent smell that is not easy to clean especially in winter. Well, you can deal with that menace with 3% hydrogen peroxide to keep it fresh and clean. Sometimes bedding used by sick folk is stained with lots of body fluids.

Hydrogen peroxide spray will do the trick as well. For decades now, hospitals have used 3% hydrogen peroxide to sterilize their bedding and mattresses. In case the mattress has a pungent scent, all you need to do is to spray it or soak it in 3% hydrogen peroxide solution and dry it in the sun, you will not need to wash. Visibly, hydrogen peroxide is the wonder chemical when it comes to bedding especially with kids around the house.

Put it in your dish water

At home, you may want to use hydrogen peroxide in your dish water to make the dishes clean faster. The hydrogen peroxide will also deal with the smell so feel free to use it generously. Any microbes operating inside the dishes and especially wooden dishes will be quickly done away with a capful of 3% hydrogen peroxide. In case you have left the dishes for ages before washing them, smile because hydrogen peroxide will rescue you from the smell of dirty dishes too. It is all in the bacteria and mold remember.

Sanitize the bathroom

The bathroom is a great place to start when cleaning the house. The bad thing is that most of the times, you will need six or so different chemicals to clean up everything. Well, this week, try out hydrogen peroxide, the multipurpose cleaner for the bowl, sink, blinds, glass, counters and all surfaces. Hydrogen peroxide will enable you to narrow down on the stuff you have to buy and also get rid of pungent chemical smells forever from your bathroom. No mold or algae will survive hydrogen peroxide, so go ahead, try it out and thank me later.

Remove household mold using the spray

As mentioned before, mold is probably one of the most hated microbes in the home. As long as there is a damp feeling in a random corner of your home, mold will show up. Hydrogen peroxide is specially suited to deal with mold in a span of time. All you need to do is to spray a 5% solution of hydrogen peroxide to the affected areas and give it half an hour. The mold will die instantly at the spraying of hydrogen peroxide, so just sweep away the residue for a permanent solution.

Use it in your swimming pool

Finally, you can use hydrogen peroxide in your swimming pool. Most pools are predisposed to accumulate algae or other microbes on the basis of their proximity to stagnant water. This can be a dangerous predisposition that encourages pest infestation as well as diseases in the pool. In the past, pool professionals have used chlorine to deal with algae and microorganisms found in the pool, which has great results. The drawback though is the fact that chlorine always produces a pungent smell, often discouraging the fun you always like to have in the pool.

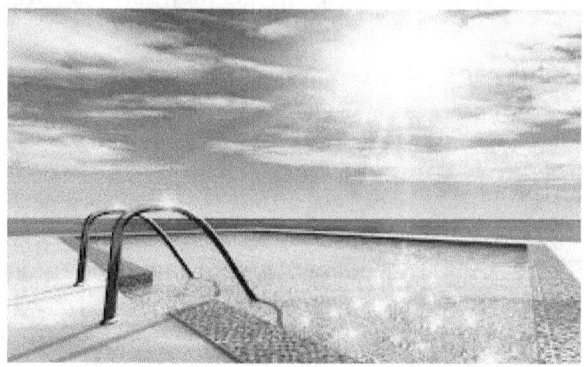

Well you can switch to using hydrogen peroxide on the swimming pool water instead. The effect will be twofold. First, the pool will be clean of any microbial activity and without chlorine stench. Secondly, you will actually be swimming in a healing bath. How awesome! The small dose that hydrogen peroxide will give you every time you go swimming will help your skin deal with acne and your body deal with fungus or pubic yeast infections. Now that is one more reason to change your swimming pool cleaning mechanism!

6. Personal Care

Personal care is a wide topic. It involves taking care of your body in the best way possible, often with a myriad of chemical applications or routine procedures that minimize the occurrence of disease. Below are ways in which hydrogen peroxide therapy will revolutionize your personal care life.

Detoxify your bath with hydrogen peroxide

As explained beforehand, hydrogen peroxide has awesome qualities that will ensure elimination of many germs in your home. To make an awesome mix of germicidal bath water, pour a quart of 3% hydrogen peroxide for every tub of warm water and soak for at least 30 minutes. In the end you will have the cleaning effect of hydrogen peroxide and your body will not suffer any skin disease attack.

Cure your foot fungus

In case you have fungus on your feet, simply spray a 50: 50 mixture of hydrogen peroxide and water and let it dry naturally. Do this daily and within a week the fungus should clear. It is just as simple as that, you don't need to do anything else or wait for weeks for the fungi to clear.

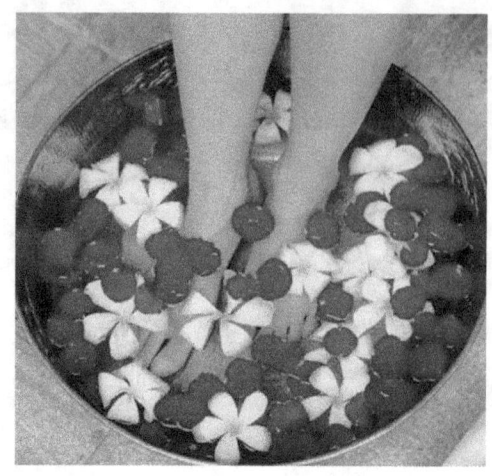

Deal with vaginal douche

For the ladies with pubic yeast infections, hydrogen peroxide may come in handy. All you will need is to add 2 cups of 3% hydrogen peroxide in a bath of water twice each week. Use this solution to douche out even chronic yeast infections by bathing for at least 30 minutes daily. You can put on relaxing music and light scented candles if you want motivation to stay longer than 30 minutes.

Dissolve your ear wax

You can use 3% hydrogen peroxide to actually dissolve your body wax in your ears. This will also serve to cleanse your ear cavity from secondary infection. Do not use it however if you have had previous infections or if you have fresh wounds in your ear. Avoid using this therapy in case you are about to fly. Finally, the hydrogen peroxide used must always be of 3% or less concentration.

Clean your contacts

If you have sensitive eyes, a 3% solution of hydrogen peroxide will effectively clean the dirt and proteins that build up on contact lenses. Removing this without a scrub will both preserve your contacts while keeping your vision awesome. The hydrogen peroxide will save you the agony of scrubbing your contacts so why not try it today. Stick to the solution at 3% since some lenses are made with very sensitive PVC.

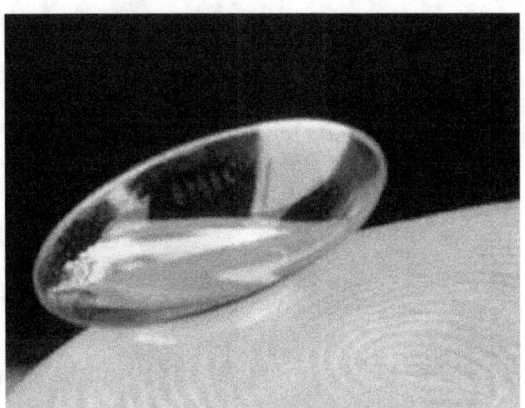

Use it for hand wash

Many medical experts support the use of hydrogen peroxide as hand wash. Actually, it is used in operation theatres to clean up during surgery. To reduce induced illnesses spread by contact and infected hands, you can dilute a wash to be by using or mixing it with soap. The diluted one is used directly on your hand wash basin or bath water. The second method is however the best. Simply mix it with your hand wash soap. The resulting solution will not only be a great soap, but an awesome disinfectant that is effective and strong.

7. Beauty

Hydrogen peroxide can easily be used to improve appearance through several body procedures. Most of the conditions addressed by hydrogen peroxide involve skin infection handling. Below are some major ways to capitalize hydrogen peroxide to improve beauty.

Use hydrogen peroxide to bleach your blonde hair

Hair can be bleached using hydrogen peroxide. The protein that is found in human hair called keratin has pigments that respond to oxidative bleaching. Simply dilute 3% hydrogen peroxide with water and expose it to your hair. You can choose to spray directly or to soak the hair in a solution. Unlike the hair dye packages, the tinge of your hair will remain natural and permanent.

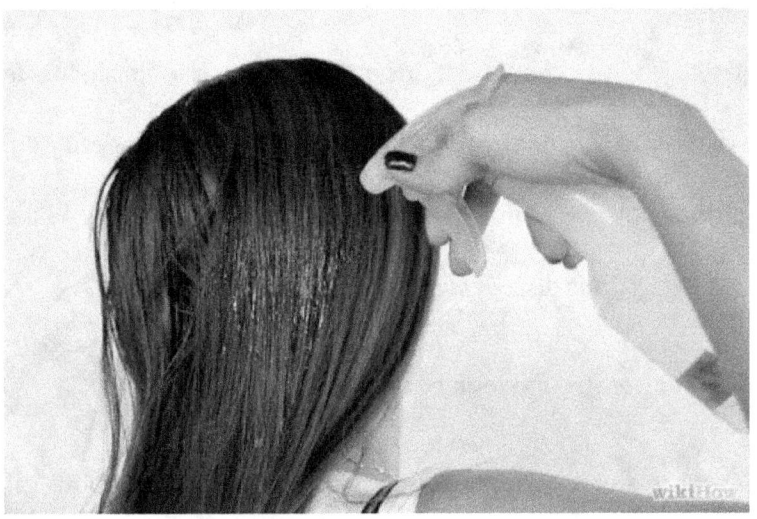

Another advantage of hydrogen peroxide bleaching is that the fading is gradual and not rapid. This gives you the chance to control the shade of bleaching you want. Hydrogen peroxide can also be used to remove yellow strands from naturally white hair, in the same procedure. Another common method of using hydrogen peroxide to bleach the hair is by mixing it with ammonium hydroxide. The mixture is fairly stable and can be used even for children.

Get rid of acne using hydrogen peroxide

In case your skin has multiple sores and acne, you may be in for a surprise. Simply dab 3% hydrogen peroxide onto the base of each acne mark and keep doing it for a week or so. Make sure you do it several times each day. The result is that your skin will be sanitized every time you clean. This in the end will lead to lower infections and a smooth skin finish. In a few days, the acne will disappear completely leaving your old smooth skin intact. Washing your face with weak hydrogen peroxide solution will also clear up dead cells thus discouraging aging and wrinkling.

Deal with skin diseases and look better

Skin diseases are either caused by fungi, bacteria or viral infection. This can be minimized by sanitizing the skin evenly each time with hydrogen peroxide washes. In the end, rash and other forms of infection will simply die down leaving your skin smooth.

8. Health

There are many health applications of hydrogen peroxide. Below are some proven ways your health can improve through application of hydrogen peroxide therapy.

Deal with colonic and enema

In case you have colonic infection or enema, you can ingest controlled versions of hydrogen peroxide to kill excess microbes. Remember hydrogen peroxide emits oxygen as a byproduct thus potentially destroying a good portion of anaerobic microbes in the colon. Simply place a cup of 3% hydrogen peroxide to 5 gallons of water for a colonic treatment. Take at least three glasses daily. For enema therapy, add 3% hydrogen peroxide to warm distilled water, one quart. You should take two glasses each day for this one. Though peroxide therapy will not fully eliminate the condition, the relief will be worth it, considering you have nothing to lose.

Use hydrogen peroxide to whiten and clean your teeth

The healing properties of hydrogen peroxide can do wonders to your teeth. You can use it to make an effective toothpaste, mouthwash, soothe a toothache or as a toothbrush cleanser. Simply take a capful of 3% hydrogen peroxide and hold it in your mouth for several minutes, preferably ten, gurgle and spit it out. In a short while you will have neither sores on your teeth, nor stains. Your teeth will glow whiter each time you do this. This is great if you have tarred teeth from drinking coffee or smoking tobacco.

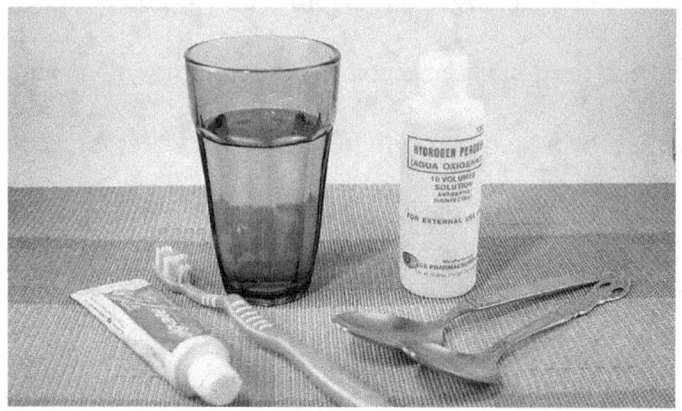

To make your own regular mouth wash, add 3% hydrogen peroxide to a dash of liquid chlorophyll. Use it regularly for awesome results. This is a very cheap solution to have, unfortunately, it could make the pharmaceutical industry lose billions in revenue so that is why people don't know about it. To make your own toothpaste, mix 3% hydrogen peroxide with baking soda to form an even paste. This paste will have the scouring properties of baking soda as well as the cleansing qualities of hydrogen peroxide, making it the ideal toothpaste for your teeth.

To get rid of toothache and evade dental procedures such as root canal and teeth removal, simply use a hydrogen peroxide mouthwash regularly. It is antifungal, antibacterial and will rid the pain in a short time when used regularly. You may alternate the use with coconut oil to completely heal your teeth.

Treat fresh wounds

Hydrogen peroxide can be used to heal wounds. A word of caution though, do not froth out your cells blindly! Dilute the hydrogen peroxide into a mild solution of around 3%. Soak the wound for about five minutes and leave to dry. Do this several times in the day. Also remember that half a bottle of hydrogen peroxide in your bath will rid you of boils, fungus and skin infections. However, cleaning of deep wounds with hydrogen peroxide is not recommended. H_2O_2 is highly oxidizing and for this reason is prone to destroy newly formed body cells, which encourages slow healing, leading to a possibility of more infection.

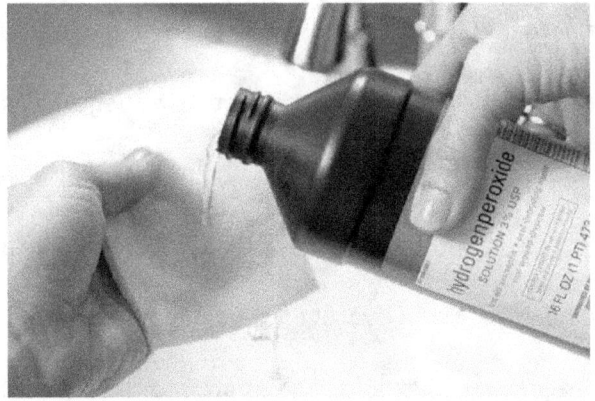

Use for nasal infections

For nose infections and wounds, use a 3% tablespoon of hydrogen peroxide, added to a cup of non-chlorinated water. This will serve as a great cure for nasal infections when sprayed directly into the nose.

9. Food Preparation

Hydrogen peroxide is generally used in the industries to sanitize food packaging and food in general. At home, you can use food grade hydrogen peroxide to achieve the same purpose but on a smaller scale. You may use it to make your food better in these ways.

Use Hydrogen To Sanitize Your Vegetables

In case you are not sure your veggies are clean, it is good to confirm it by using hydrogen peroxide. Simply use 3% hydrogen peroxide solution to soak them and add a little warm water to soothe the vegetables. Leave them intact for close to ten minutes and drain. In the end, the vegetables will be thoroughly clean and they will definitely last longer in case of refrigeration. A combination of hydrogen peroxide and vinegar is the perfect cleaning agent for fruits and veggies around the kitchen.

Sanitize Your Meat Before Cooking

Meat can have potentially dangerous mold or microbes on the edges when stored for a long time. This includes even refrigerated meat. For this reason, the surface can be sanitized; just to be sure you are having healthy food. Do this in the last five minutes of cooking it so that it can drain. All you will need is a very mild hydrogen peroxide solution, probably 1%.

Preserve Leftover Salads

If your veggie or fruit salad has been left over, no problem! You can still have it the following day by slowing down the decomposition process. Eliminate all the bacteria and molds by simply spraying a thin layer of hydrogen peroxide directly on it and covering with a clear foil or glass cover. Refrigerate it after this for the best results. It will still be fresh the following morning.

Marinade Your Meat To Make It Softer

Sometimes, your meat is best cooked tender. What you may not have is the fuel to keep cooking it or the patience to wait. In that case, you can place your meat in a solution of hydrogen peroxide and warm water. Allow it to soak for at least one hour. When cooked, the meat will be very tender. It will also be slightly bleached so you may consider adding some food color. Finally, you can use hydrogen peroxide as a sterilizing agent for food packaging materials.

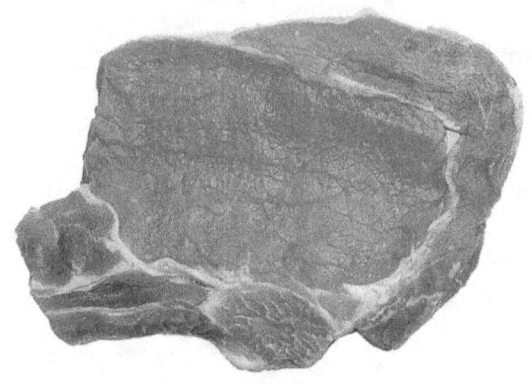

10.   Other Uses for Hydrogen Peroxide

Around the home, the atmosphere is often a myriad of tasks that need to be done. The efficiency of hydrogen peroxide has not shied away from some of the weirdest tasks around the home. It can actually be used in the following ways with some awesome results.

Get Rid Of Mites With Hydrogen Peroxide

Getting rid of mites in the home can be a daunting dilemma. On one hand the small army of destructors will paralyze your happiness. On the other hand, most of the pesticides designed to fight them off are dangerous chemicals that you may not want to see near your home. Well, you can use hydrogen peroxide to deal with them once and for all. Simply spray a thin solution of 3% hydrogen peroxide on the skin of a mite infested person, garment or animal. The mites will fall off dead instantly.

Germinate seeds in the home

For faster germination of seeds, use hydrogen peroxide to activate the seed enzymes and also to break the seed scars of hardy seeds. Seeds that take up to a month to germinate can do so in just days under careful use of hydrogen peroxide. Simply soak the seeds in 6% hydrogen peroxide for a reasonable period of time. You can try an experimental seed as different seeds will take different lengths of time to germinate under influence of hydrogen peroxide. This is mainly due to the fact that they have different structures. Wheatgrass seeds should be soaked for only thirty minutes and planted. They will take five days to mature instead of seven!

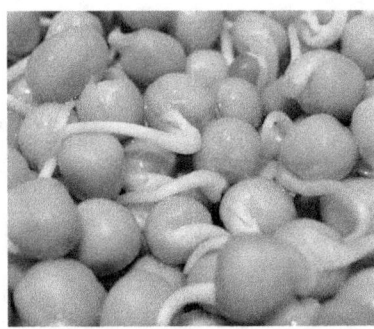

Use Hydrogen Peroxide On Pets

Apart from disinfecting their food and environment, hydrogen peroxide can deworm pets if placed in minute quantities in their drinking water. Dogs will generally appreciate the gesture and stay worm-free thus keeping them happy and healthy. Cats and dogs hate conventional medicine and vaccines and de-wormers, so you can try this awesome alternative to keep them happy. You may also clean their litter and pillows using a spray of hydrogen peroxide to kill off pests and keep the smell down. Using ammonia to clean really confuses pets. Remember, dogs and cats know how to mark their territory with urine and it is very easy to imagine their territory has been invaded since ammonia generally smells like urine so your dog and cat will hate it too.

11.   Conclusion

No matter how you may choose to use it, it is very clear hydrogen peroxide will leave your home fresh, your body healthy and your family happy. The many unique features of hydrogen peroxide make it the best choice for home care, way above board of the safety standards you must keep at home. Below are some of the key benefits of using hydrogen peroxide that will make you want to keep using it indefinitely.

First, remember hydrogen peroxide is anti-viral, anti-bacterial, anti-mildew and anti-mold! Now that is a heavy package in just one agent. Most of the products you will find around in the market will either offer one thing or leave out the other. For instance, you will need to buy at least three different chemical cleansers to deal with viruses, bacteria, mildew, algae and mold. Be happy you have discovered hydrogen peroxide, and the budget is unbelievable.

It is also great to know that hydrogen peroxide is not toxic to people, to the environment or to the plants. Most of the alternative chemicals we use daily in our homes have huge question marks as far as safety is concerned. For instance, most anti-viral medications are inherently harmful to the environment and may contain heavy metals thus compounding the problem. Hydrogen peroxide is simply oxygen and water. How awesome.

Since hydrogen peroxide is multipurpose, you will not need to buy many products. It will save you the need to buy many different types of cleaners and cleaning agents thus significantly cutting your budget. Another factor that will keep you loving hydrogen peroxide is that it is very cheap to buy. Simply buy in bulk and dilute on the go according to your need. Even the 'expensive' food grade hydrogen peroxide is not as expensive as some cleaning agents around the home.

Finally, whether you use it to bathe, to wash or to clean the house, it will keep your sponges, scrubbers and cleaning tools a lot cleaner. Hydrogen peroxide actually disinfects them in the process every time you use them to clean anything, thus maintaining a healthy home.

There are tons of things to love about using hydrogen peroxide therapy in your body and home. The beauty of keeping on its use is the assurance that your huge savings on budget also mean a longer and healthier life for you. At the end of the day, your greatest utility out of any product is the

peace of mind it gives you.

Enjoy this book?

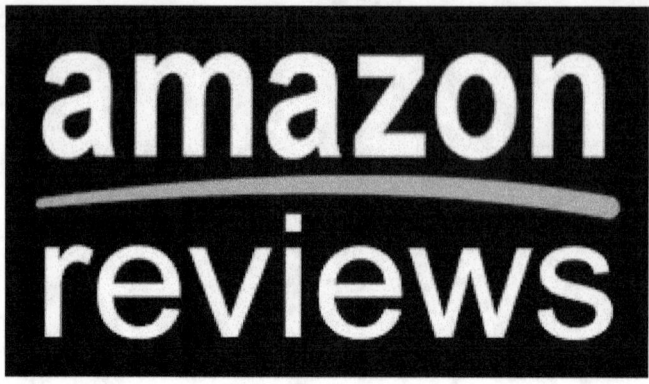

Please leave an Amazon review below and let me know what you liked about this book as that would help a self-published author such as myself a great deal. Thank you!

Please leave a review at the following book URL:
http://amzn.com/B00P5AB1EE

www.ingramcontent.com/pod-product-compliance
Lightning Source LLC
Chambersburg PA
CBHW071342310526
45790CB00018B/1081